28 Days Of
Chair Yoga For Senior's

How to Stay Strong, Flexible, and Happy in Your Senior Years

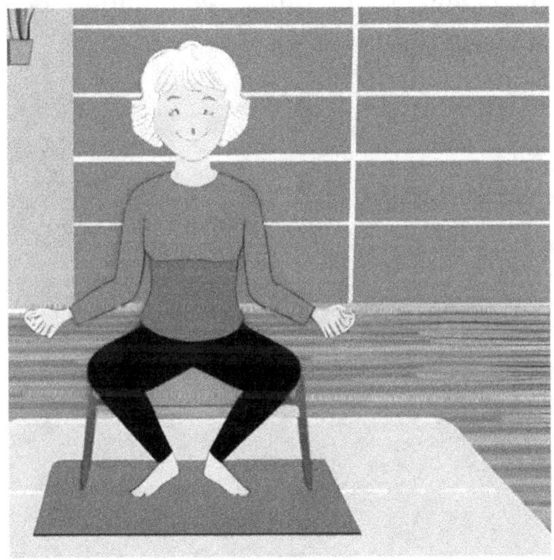

Lana Cochran

2 Copyright Material

3 Copyright Material

4 Copyright Material

5 Copyright Material

Chapter 1: The Benefits of Chair Yoga

The benefits of chair yoga are numerous and encompass physical, mental, and emotional well-being. Chair yoga offers a host of benefits specifically tailored to seniors, making it an ideal practice for maintaining and enhancing their overall well-being

Understanding the Advantages

1. **Physical Well-Being**: Chair yoga is an exceptional avenue for seniors to maintain and improve physical well-being. The gentle, supported poses help enhance flexibility, range of motion, and joint health. Through regular practice, you can expect to experience increased vitality and reduced stiffness in your body.

2. **Mind-Body Connection**: One of the core principles of yoga is the mind-body connection. Chair yoga encourages this connection through conscious breath awareness and mindful movement. By cultivating this awareness, you can manage stress, improve focus, and promote relaxation, leading to a more balanced and harmonious life.

3. **Functional Strength**: Engaging in chair yoga regularly promotes functional strength, the kind that supports your daily activities and enhances your independence. As you progress, you will notice improved muscle tone and stability, which contribute to better posture and overall strength.

4. **Pain Management**: For those dealing with chronic pain or discomfort, chair yoga offers a gentle yet effective way to alleviate symptoms. The supportive nature of the practice helps relieve tension, reduce pain, and enhance the body's natural healing processes.

5. **Cardiovascular Health**: The controlled breathing techniques utilized in chair yoga have a positive impact on cardiovascular health. By practicing mindful breathwork, you can improve circulation, lower blood pressure, and contribute to a healthier heart.

Integrating Chair Yoga into Your Routine

Practical Tips

- **Start Slowly**: If you are new to yoga or have physical limitations, begin with shorter sessions, and gradually increase the duration as you become more comfortable.

- **Consistency is Key**: Aim for a consistent practice, even if it is just a few minutes a day. Consistency is more important than intensity.

- **Listen to Your Body**: Honor your body's signals. If a pose feels uncomfortable or painful, modify it or skip it altogether. Your comfort and safety are paramount.

- **Use Props**: Embrace the use of props such as blankets, blocks, and straps to enhance your practice and provide additional support.

Step-by-Step Instructions: Breath Awareness

1. **Find a Comfortable Seat**: Sit upright in a sturdy chair with your feet flat on the floor, hip-width apart. Rest your hands on your thighs.

2. **Close Your Eyes**: Gently close your eyes, allowing your awareness to turn inward.

3. **Deepen Your Breath**: Inhale deeply through your nose, feeling your abdomen expand. Exhale slowly and completely through your mouth.

4. **Count Your Breath**: Inhale for a count of four, then exhale for a count of six. Focus on making your exhales longer than your inhales, promoting relaxation.

5. **Observe Your Breath**: Notice the sensation of your breath as it flows in and out. Let go of any tension with each exhale.

6. **Stay Present**: If your mind starts to wander, gently bring your attention back to your breath. Continue this breath awareness for 5-10 minutes.

As you wrap up this chapter, take a moment to reflect on the potential that chair yoga holds for your well-being. By understanding its benefits and integrating simple practices like breath awareness into your daily routine, you are laying the foundation for a journey of strength, flexibility, and happiness in your senior years. In the next chapter, we will guide you through creating a comfortable and safe space for your chair yoga practice.

Chapter 2: Setting Up Your Practice Space

Welcome to Chapter 2 of "28 Days of Chair Yoga for Seniors." In this chapter, we will delve into the essential aspects of creating a conducive practice space for your chair yoga journey. As an experienced yoga instructor with over 25 years of expertise, I am here to guide you through the process of setting up your environment to ensure comfort, safety, and optimal support.

Creating Comfort

Creating a comfortable space is crucial for an enjoyable and effective chair yoga practice. Here is how you can ensure your comfort:

Practical Tips

1. **Choose a Quiet Area**: Find a quiet and peaceful corner of your home where you can practice without distractions. This will help you focus and immerse yourself in your practice.

2. **Use Soft Lighting**: Natural light is ideal, but if that is not possible, opt for soft, diffused lighting that is easy on the eyes. Avoid harsh, direct lighting.

3. **Temperature Control**: Maintain a comfortable room temperature. If needed, have a blanket nearby to keep you warm during relaxation poses.

Step-by-Step Instructions: Creating a Relaxing Ambiance

1. **Clear the Space**: Remove any clutter or obstacles from your practice area to create a clean and inviting space.

2. **Add Personal Touches**: Place items that bring you joy and calmness nearby, such as a favorite plant, soothing artwork, or a scented candle.

3. **Set an Intention**: Take a moment to set a positive intention for your practice. This could be a word, phrase, or feeling that resonates with you.

Choosing the Right Chair and Props

Selecting the appropriate chair and props is essential for ensuring optimal support during your chair yoga practice.

Practical Tips

1. **Sturdy Chair**: Choose a stable, armless chair with a firm seat and backrest. Avoid chairs with wheels or swivels.

2. **Seat Height:** Select a chair that allows you to sit with your feet flat on the floor and your knees at a 90-degree angle. You may use cushions or folded blankets to adjust the seat height if needed.

3. **Props for Support**: Keep a few yoga props handy, such as blocks, blankets, and straps. These can enhance your practice and provide additional support in various poses.

Step-by-Step Instructions: Choosing the Right Chair and Props

1. **Chair Selection**: Test different chairs in your home to find one that offers stability and comfort. The chair should support your weight without wobbling.

2. **Seat Height Adjustment**: Sit in the chair and ensure your feet are flat on the floor. If your feet dangle, place cushions or folded blankets under them until your knees are at a comfortable 90-degree angle.

3. **Props Placement**: Arrange your props within arm's reach, so you can easily access them during your practice. For example, place blocks on the floor beside your chair and have a folded blanket nearby for additional cushioning.

Alignment and Posture

Proper alignment and posture are fundamental in chair yoga to prevent strain and injury.

Practical Tips:

1. **Sit Upright**: Align your head, shoulders, and hips while sitting in the chair. Avoid slouching or leaning too far forward.

2. **Engage Your Core**: Gently engage your core muscles to support your spine and maintain stability.

Step-by-Step Instructions: Finding Optimal Alignment

1. **Sit at the Front of the Chair**: Position yourself so that your sitting bones are near the front edge of the chair. This allows you to maintain a natural curve in your lower back.

2. **Feet Placement**: Keep your feet hip-width apart and parallel. Ensure your knees are aligned with your ankles and pointing straight ahead.

3. **Spinal Alignment**: Lengthen your spine upward while allowing your shoulders to relax. Imagine a gentle lift from the crown of your head.

4. **Relax Your Shoulders**: Soften your shoulder blades down your back. Let your arms hang comfortably by your sides or rest them on your thighs.

As you complete this chapter, take a moment to appreciate the effort you have put into creating a nurturing space for your chair yoga practice. The environment you have set up will support your journey toward strength, flexibility, and happiness in your senior years. In the next chapter, we will explore the profound benefits of breath and mindfulness in chair yoga.

Breath and Mindfulness

Welcome to Chapter 3 of "28 Days of Chair Yoga for Seniors." In this chapter, we will explore the profound connection between breath and mindfulness in chair yoga. As an experienced yoga instructor with over 25 years of practice, I am thrilled to guide you through the transformative journey of breath awareness and mindfulness techniques to enhance your well-being.

The Power of Breath Awareness

Breath awareness is a cornerstone of yoga practice. It not only calms the mind but also supports the body's natural rhythms and processes.

Practical Tips

1. **Conscious Breathing**: Throughout your chair yoga practice, cultivate awareness of your breath. Breathe naturally and observe the sensation of each inhalation and exhalation.

2. **Diaphragmatic Breathing**: Practice diaphragmatic breathing by allowing your abdomen to expand on inhale and contract on exhale. This deepens your breath and promotes relaxation.

3. **Counting Breath**: Use a simple counting technique: Inhale for a count of four and exhale for a count of six. Adjust the counts to a pace that feels comfortable for you.

Mindfulness Techniques for Stress Reduction

Mindfulness involves being fully present in the moment. Incorporating mindfulness techniques into your chair yoga practice can reduce stress and enhance your focus.

Practical Tips

1. **Body Scan**: Scan your body from head to toe, bringing awareness to each area. Notice any sensations, tension, or relaxation you experience.

2. **Focused Attention**: During your practice, focus your attention on the sensations of movement, breath, and the alignment of your body. This helps anchor you in the present moment.

3. **Mindful Observation**: Choose an object in your practice space—a plant, a candle, or an artwork. Gently observe its details, colors, and textures, allowing your mind to find stillness.

Step-by-Step Breath-Centered Chair Yoga Sequences

Incorporating breath-centered chair yoga sequences into your practice enhances the mind-body connection and amplifies the benefits of yoga.

Practical Tips

1. **Seated Mountain Pose with Breath**: Sit comfortably in your chair. Inhale, lengthening your spine, and raising your arms overhead. Exhale, bringing your hands to the heart center. Repeat for 5-8 breaths.

2. **Seated Cat-Cow Breath**: Inhale, arch your back and lift your chest (cow). Exhale, round your spine and drop your chin (cat). Repeat for 6-10 cycles.

3. **Seated Twist with Breath**: Inhale, lengthen your spine. Exhale, turn to the right, place your left hand on your right thigh and your right hand on the back of the chair. Inhale to center, exhale to twist left. Repeat for 3-5 breaths on each side.

4. **Mindful Relaxation**: Sit back comfortably in your chair, close your eyes, and focus on your breath. Inhale deeply for a count of four, exhale for a count of six. With each exhale, release tension from your body. Continue for 5-10 minutes.

Step-by-Step Instructions: Seated Mountain Pose with Breath

1. **Sit Tall**: Sit near the edge of your chair, feet flat on the floor, and hands resting on your thighs.

2. **Inhale and Extend**: Inhale, lengthen your spine, and reach your arms overhead. Feel the stretch in your sides and the lift of your chest.

3. **Exhale and Center**: Exhale, bring your hands to heart center in a prayer position. Feel the grounding energy as your hands meet.

4. **Repeat**: Inhale, extend your arms overhead, and exhale, bringing your hands to the heart center. Continue this movement with your breath for 5-8 rounds.

As you conclude this chapter, take a moment to appreciate the tranquility that breath awareness and mindfulness bring to your chair yoga practice. By incorporating these techniques, you are nurturing a sense of calm, focus, and presence. In the upcoming chapter, we will explore gentle warm-up exercises to prepare your body for deeper stretches and poses

Chapter 4: Gentle Warm-Up Exercises

Greetings and welcome to Chapter 4 of "28 Days of Chair Yoga for Seniors." In this chapter, we will dive into the art of gentle warm-up exercises – the essential foundation for preparing your body and joints for deeper stretches and poses. As a seasoned yoga instructor with over 25 years of practice, I am delighted to guide you through a series of mindful movements that will invigorate your body and set the stage for a rewarding practice.

The Importance of Warm-Up

Warming up is crucial to ensure the safety and effectiveness of your chair yoga practice. Gentle movements help increase blood flow, loosen muscles, and improve joint mobility.

Practical Tips

1. **Gradual Progression**: Begin with gentle movements and gradually increase the intensity. Allow your body time to adapt and open up.

2. **Mindful Movement**: Approach your warm-up with mindfulness. Focus on each movement and its effects on your body.

3. **Breath Connection**: Sync your breath with your movements. Inhale as you lengthen or expand, and exhale as you contract or release.

Preparing for Deeper Poses

A proper warm-up prepares your body for deeper stretches and poses. It enhances flexibility, reduces the risk of injury, and helps you move more freely.

Practical Tips

1. **Target Different Areas**: Include movements that target various parts of your body – neck, shoulders, spine, hips, and legs.

2. **Fluidity**: Create a flow in your warm-up routine. Transition from one movement to another with grace and intention.

3. **Mind-Body Connection**: As you move, bring your awareness to the sensations in your body. Notice areas that may feel tight or tense.

Modifications and Variations

Adapting warm-up exercises to suit your mobility level is essential. Explore variations that provide the right amount of challenge without causing strain.

Practical Tips

1. **Listen to Your Body**: Choose variations that feel comfortable and accessible. If a movement causes discomfort, modify it, or skip it.

2. **Chair Support**: Use the chair for added stability. Hold onto the backrest or seat for balance during certain movements.

3. **Range of Motion**: If you have limited mobility, focus on gentle, smaller movements that gradually increase your range over time.

Step-by-Step Instructions: Neck and Shoulder Warm-Up

1. **1. Sit Tall:** Sit at the edge of your chair, feet flat on the floor, and hands on your feet. Allow your hands to rest on your thighs.

2. **Neck Tilt (Ear to Shoulder)**:

    - Inhale, lengthen your spine.

    - Exhale, gently drop your right ear toward your right shoulder.

    - Inhale, return to center.

    - Exhale, tilt your left ear toward your left shoulder.

    - Repeat for 3-5 rounds on each side.

3. **Shoulder Rolls**:

    - Inhale, lift your shoulders toward your ears.

    - Exhale, roll your shoulders back and down.

    - Inhale, lift your shoulders again.

    - Exhale, roll them forward and down.

    - Repeat for 6-8 rounds.

4. **Arm Swings**:

- Inhale, reach your arms forward.

- Exhale, swing your arms out to the sides and back.

- Inhale, bring your arms back to the center.

- Exhale, lower your arms.

- Repeat for 6-8 rounds.

5. **Seated Spinal Twist**:

- Inhale, sit tall.

- Exhale and twist your torso to the right, resting your left hand on the outside of your right leg and your right hand on the chair's back. Inhale to center.

- Exhale, twist to the left.

- Repeat for 3-5 rounds on each side.

As you conclude this chapter, acknowledge the gentle warmth you have cultivated in your body. By embracing these warm-up exercises, you are priming yourself for deeper poses and greater flexibility. In the upcoming chapter, we will explore seated forward bends and backbends to enhance spinal flexibility and posture.

Chapter 5: Seated Forward Bends and Backbends

Welcome to Chapter 5 of "28 Days of Chair Yoga for Seniors." In this chapter, we will embark on a journey of seated forward bends and gentle backbends – a delightful exploration that enhances spinal flexibility, improves posture, and contributes to your overall well-being. Drawing upon my 25 years of yoga expertise, I am excited to guide you through these transformative poses with care and precision.

Seated Forward Bends for Spinal Flexibility

Seated forward bends offer a wonderful opportunity to lengthen and stretch your spine, promoting flexibility and relaxation.

Practical Tips

1. **Slow and Steady**: Approach forward bends with a gentle and patient mindset. Avoid forcing yourself into a deep stretch.

2. **Breathe into the Stretch**: Inhale as you lengthen your spine, and exhale as you fold forward. Use your breath to deepen the stretch gradually.

3. **Support with Props**: If your hands do not reach your feet, use a strap or a towel around your feet for support.

Gentle Backbends for Improved Posture

Gentle backbends are beneficial for counteracting the effects of sitting and improving posture.

Practical Tips

1. **Engage Your Core**: As you move into a gentle backbend, engage your core muscles to support your spine.

2. **Avoid Compression**: Ensure that you are not compressing your lower back. Focus on creating length and space in your spine.

3. **Use the Chair for Support**: The back of the chair can provide support as you lean back into your backbend.

Tips for Ensuring Proper Alignment and Preventing Discomfort

Maintaining proper alignment is crucial to ensure the safety and effectiveness of your forward bends and backbends.

Practical Tips

1. **Spinal Alignment**: In forward bends, hinge from your hips while keeping your spine long. Avoid rounding your back.

2. **Engage Muscles**: Engage your core and back muscles to support your spine in the backbends. This reduces strain on your lower back.

3. **Modify as Needed**: If you have limited flexibility or mobility, adapt the poses to your comfort level. Use props and gentle movements to ease into the poses.

Step-by-Step Instructions: Seated Forward Bend and Supported Backbend

1. **Seated Forward Bend**:

    - Sit tall at the edge of your chair, feet flat on the floor.

    - Inhale, lengthen your spine.

    - Exhale, hinge forward from your hips, leading with your chest.

    - Place your hands on your shins, ankles, or feet, depending on your flexibility.

    - Inhale, lengthen your spine again.

    - Exhale, deepen the forward fold, maintaining a long spine.

    - Hold for 3-5 breaths.

    - To release, inhale and slowly move back to an upright position.

2. **Supported Backbend**:

    - Sit tall, placing your hands on the back of the chair for support.

    - Inhale, lengthen your spine.

- Exhale, gently arch your upper back, drawing your shoulder blades together.

- Look upward without straining your neck.

- Inhale, maintaining the arch in your upper back.

- Exhale, release the backbend and sit upright.

- Repeat for 3-5 rounds, focusing on opening your chest and heart center.

As you conclude this chapter, recognize the positive impact that seated forward bends and gentle backbends can have on your spinal health and posture. With mindful practice and attention to alignment, you are nurturing your body's strength and flexibility. In the upcoming chapter, we will delve into the benefits of seated twists and spinal mobility for your overall well-being.

Chapter 6: Twists and Spinal Mobility

Greetings and welcome to Chapter 6 of "28 Days of Chair Yoga for Seniors." In this chapter, we will embark on an exploration of seated twists and their profound impact on spinal health, flexibility, digestion, and circulation. Drawing upon my extensive experience as a yoga instructor of over 25 years, I am excited to guide you through the art of twisting poses, helping you unlock the benefits they offer for your overall well-being.

The Art of Seated Twists

Seated twists are a gentle yet potent way to enhance spinal mobility and promote a healthy range of motion.

Practical Tips

1. **Alignment Matters**: Begin with a solid foundation. Ensure your feet are grounded and your sitting bones are firmly on the chair.

2. **Engage the Core**: Engaging your core muscles provides stability and supports your spine as you twist.

3. **Breathe into the Twist**: Inhale to lengthen your spine, and exhale as you deepen the twist. Use your breath to create space and openness.

Benefits of Twisting Poses

Twisting poses offer a range of benefits, including improved digestion, enhanced circulation, and a sense of renewal.

1. **Aid Digestion**: Twists stimulate the abdominal organs, aiding digestion and promoting detoxification.

2. **Enhance Circulation**: Twisting compresses and then releases the internal organs, increasing blood flow and oxygenation.

3. **Energize and Renew**: Twists create a gentle massage for the spine, promoting relaxation and revitalization.

Gradually Deepen Your Twist Practice

As with any yoga practice, gradual progression is key. Approach deepening your twist practice with patience and awareness.

Practical Tips

1. **Start Small**: Begin with gentle twists and gradually increase the depth over time as your body becomes more comfortable.

2. **Listen to Your Body**: Take note of your body's signals. If you feel discomfort or strain, ease out of the pose, or reduce the twist.

3. **Prop Support**: If needed, use a prop like a pillow or cushion to support your knees or hips during twists.

Step-by-Step Instructions: Seated Chair Twist

1. **Sit Tall**: Sit at the edge of your chair, feet flat on the floor, and hands on your thighs.

2. **Inhale and Lengthen**: Inhale, lengthen your spine upward, imagining a gentle lift from the crown of your head.

3. **Exhale and Twist**: Exhale, slowly twist your torso to the right. Place your left hand on the outside of your right thigh and your right hand on the backrest of the chair.

4. **Breathe and Release**: Inhale, find length in your spine. Exhale, deepen the twist slightly. Feel the gentle compression in your abdomen.

5. **Maintain for a Few Breaths**: Hold the twist for 3-5 breaths, maintaining a steady breath and soft gaze.

6. **Inhale and Unwind**: Inhale, return to center, and exhale to release the twist.

7. **Repeat on the Other Side**: Mirror the twist by placing your right hand on your left thigh and your left hand on the backrest. Hold for 3-5 breaths.

As you conclude this chapter, appreciate the newfound freedom and vitality that seated twists offer to your spine and internal organs. By embracing these poses mindfully and gradually deepening your practice, you are nurturing your body's resilience and supporting its natural functions. In the upcoming chapter, we will delve into hip and leg mobility, exploring poses that enhance flexibility and ease discomfort.

Chapter 7: Hip and Leg Mobility

Welcome to Chapter 7 of "28 Days of Chair Yoga for Seniors." In this chapter, we will delve into the realm of hip and leg mobility, exploring the transformative power of seated poses that enhance flexibility, relieve tension, and promote overall comfort. As an experienced yoga instructor with over 25 years of practice, I am excited to guide you through a series of chair yoga poses designed to improve lower body mobility and bring a sense of ease to your hips and legs.

Section 1: Unveiling Hip and Leg Mobility

Hip and leg mobility plays a crucial role in maintaining an active and balanced lifestyle. Seated poses can provide an effective means to enhance flexibility and alleviate discomfort.

Practical Tips:

1. **Gentle Approach**: Approach hip and leg stretches with gentleness and patience. The focus is on creating space and ease, not pushing into discomfort.

2. **Mindful Breathing**: Incorporate deep, steady breaths into your poses. Inhale to lengthen, and exhale to relax and deepen the stretch.

3. **Modify as Needed**: Use props like cushions or folded blankets to support your hips and knees, allowing for a comfortable stretch.

Relieving Tension through Gentle Hip Stretches

Gentle hip stretches can provide immense relief from tension and discomfort, improving your overall mobility and well-being.

Practical Tips

1. **Consistency**: Consistently include hip stretches in your practice to gradually increase flexibility and release tension.

2. **Warm-Up**: Engage in a brief warm-up before hip stretches to prepare the muscles and joints for deeper movements.

3. **Engage Core and Breathe**: Engage your core muscles to support your spine and use your breath to guide you deeper into the stretch.

Step-by-Step Chair Yoga Poses for Lower Body Mobility

Incorporating chair yoga poses can effectively improve lower body mobility, benefiting your hips, thighs, and legs.

Practical Tips

1. **Stay Mindful**: Pay close attention to the sensations in your body as you move into each pose. If you feel any pain, back off and modify the pose.

2. **Stay Connected**: Maintain a connection between your breath and movement. Inhale to prepare, and exhale to ease into the stretch.

3. **Regular Practice**: Dedicate a few minutes each day to these poses for optimal results. Gradually, you will notice increased flexibility and reduced discomfort.

Step-by-Step Instructions: Seated Hip Opener

1. **1. Sit Upright:** Sit at the edge of your chair, feet flat on the floor, and hands on your thighs.

2. **Cross Your Ankle**: Cross your right ankle over your left knee, allowing your right knee to drop gently to the side.

3. **Lengthen Your Spine**: Inhale, lengthen your spine upward, finding a tall, proud posture.

4. **Lean Forward**: Exhale, gently hinge forward from your hips, leading with your chest. Keep your back straight and your gaze forward.

5. **Feel the Stretch**: You'll feel a gentle stretch in your right hip and outer thigh. Breathe deeply into this sensation.

6. **Hold and Breathe**: Hold the stretch for 3-5 breaths, deepening it slightly with each exhale.

7. **Release and Repeat**: Inhale, slowly come back to an upright position. Switch sides and repeat the stretch with your left ankle over your right knee.

As you conclude this chapter, acknowledge the newfound freedom and comfort you are cultivating in your hips and legs through chair yoga. By incorporating these gentle stretches into your practice and embracing mindful movement, you are enhancing your overall mobility and well-being. In the upcoming chapter, we will focus on strengthening your core, providing you with tools to improve stability and support your spine.

Chapter 8: Strengthening Your Core

Greetings and welcome to Chapter 8 of "28 Days of Chair Yoga for Seniors." In this chapter, we will delve into the significance of core strength and its role in providing stability, supporting your spine, and enhancing your overall well-being. As an experienced yoga instructor with over 25 years of practice, I am thrilled to guide you through a series of chair-based exercises that will engage and strengthen your core muscles, helping you build a foundation of strength and balance.

Embracing Core Strength for Stability

A strong core is the cornerstone of a stable and functional body. Core muscles provide support for everyday activities and help maintain proper posture.

Practical Tips

1. **Mindful Engagement**: Approach core exercises with mindfulness. Focus on activating the core muscles and maintaining proper alignment.

2. **Consistent Practice**: Dedicate a few minutes each day to core-strengthening exercises. Consistency is key to building and maintaining strength.

3. **Breath Connection**: Sync your breath with your movements. Inhale to prepare, and exhale to engage and contract your core muscles.

Chair-Based Core Exercises

Chair yoga offers a safe and effective way to strengthen your core muscles without straining your back or neck.

Practical Tips

1. **Begin with Basics**: Start with basic core exercises to establish a solid foundation before progressing to more challenging movements.

2. **Modify for Comfort**: If you experience discomfort or strain, modify the exercises, or reduce the range of motion.

3. **Quality over Quantity**: Focus on proper form and control rather than the number of repetitions. Quality movement is more effective than quantity.

Progression of Core Movements

Gradually progress from gentle core movements to more challenging variations as your strength increases.

Practical Tips

1. **Gradual Intensity**: As you become more comfortable with the basic exercises, explore variations that increase the challenge without compromising form.

2. **Mind-Body Connection**: Keep your awareness on your core muscles throughout each movement. Feel the engagement and release with each breath.

3. **Listen to Your Body**: Take note of your body's signals. If a movement causes discomfort or strain, return to a previous variation, or modify the exercise.

Step-by-Step Instructions: Seated Leg Lift with Core Activation

1. **1. Sit Tall:** Sit at the edge of your chair, feet flat on the floor, and direct your feet.

2. **Engage Your Core**: Inhale deeply and as you exhale, draw your navel towards your spine, engaging your core muscles.

3. **Lift One Leg**: Inhale, and as you exhale, lift one foot a few inches off the floor while keeping your core engaged.

4. **Hold and Breathe**: Hold the lifted leg for 3-5 breaths, maintaining core engagement. Focus on stability and balance.

5. **Lower the Leg**: Inhale as you lower the leg back down, releasing the core engagement.

6. **Alternate Sides**: Repeat the lift with the other leg, engaging your core as you lift and releasing as you lower.

As you conclude this chapter, acknowledge the progress you are making in cultivating a strong and stable core through chair-based exercises. By consistently incorporating these movements into your practice and focusing on proper alignment and engagement, you are strengthening your foundation and enhancing your overall physical well-being.

In the upcoming chapter, we will explore the benefits of balance and coordination, guiding you through poses that improve stability and enhance body awareness.

Chapter 9: Balance and Coordination

Greetings and welcome to Chapter 9 of "28 Days of Chair Yoga for Seniors." In this chapter, we will delve into the realm of balance and coordination, exploring the transformative power of chair yoga poses that enhance stability, prevent falls, and promote overall body awareness. As an experienced yoga instructor with over 25 years of practice, I am excited to guide you through a series of practical exercises and balance-focused poses that will improve your equilibrium and coordination, empowering you to move with grace and confidence.

Embracing Balance and Coordination

Balance and coordination are essential for maintaining independence and a high quality of life. Chair yoga provides a safe and effective way to enhance these crucial skills.

Practical Tips

1. **Mind-Body Connection**: Approach balance exercises with a heightened awareness of your body's movements. Focus on maintaining steady breath and alignment.

2. **Use Support**: If needed, keep the chair close by for support during balance poses. Gradually reduce reliance on the chair as you gain confidence.

3. **Daily Practice**: Dedicate a few moments each day to balance-focused exercises. Consistent practice will yield gradual improvements.

Enhancing Stability and Fall Prevention

Chair yoga offers valuable tools to improve stability and reduce the risk of falls, allowing you to move safely and confidently in your daily life.

Practical Tips

1. **Mindful Transitions**: Pay close attention to transitions between poses. Slow and deliberate movements enhance your stability.

2. **Focus on Alignment**: Maintain proper alignment to create a solid foundation. Engage your core muscles for added support.

3. **Eyes and Drishti**: Fix your gaze on a stationary point to enhance your focus and balance. A steady gaze helps stabilize your posture.

Incorporating Balance-Focused Poses

Explore a variety of chair yoga poses that enhance balance, coordination, and body awareness.

Practical Tips

1. **Start Simple**: Begin with basic balance poses before progressing to more advanced variations.

2. **Gentle Exploration**: Ease into each pose gradually, allowing your body to adapt and find its balance.

3. **Breathe and Center**: Maintain a steady breath throughout each pose. Inhale to prepare, and exhale to find stability.

Step-by-Step Instructions: Seated Tree Pose

1. **1. Sit Tall:** Sit at the edge of your chair, feet flat on the floor, and hands on your feet.

2. **Center Yourself**: Inhale deeply, feeling grounded through your sitting bones. Imagine roots extending from your feet into the earth.

3. **Shift Your Weight**: Transfer your weight onto your left foot, firmly pressing it onto the floor.

4. **Place Your Foot**: Lift your right foot off the floor, and gently place the sole of your right foot on your left inner calf or thigh. Find a position that is comfortable for you.

5. **Hands at Heart Center**: Bring your hands to heart center in a prayer position. Find a point of focus to steady your gaze.

6. **Breathe and Balance**: Hold the pose for 3-5 breaths, finding stability and balance. Engage your core muscles to support your posture.

7. **Release and Repeat**: Lower your right foot back to the floor, returning to a seated position. Switch sides and repeat the pose with your left foot on your right leg.

As you conclude this chapter, embrace the sense of empowerment that balance, and coordination bring to your chair yoga practice. By incorporating these exercises and poses mindfully and consistently, you are enhancing your stability, preventing falls, and cultivating a deeper connection between your body and mind. In the upcoming chapter, we will explore the art of relaxation and restoration, guiding you through techniques to promote calmness and rejuvenation.

Chapter 10: Relaxation and Stress Relief

Welcome to Chapter 10 of "28 Days of Chair Yoga for Seniors." In this chapter, we will explore the art of relaxation and stress relief through chair yoga, delving into guided relaxation techniques and gentle stretches that will help you unwind and cultivate a profound sense of calm and tranquility. Drawing upon my extensive experience as a yoga instructor with over 25 years of practice, I am honored to guide you through a series of practical exercises that will support your well-being by reducing stress and promoting relaxation.

Chair Yoga for Relaxation and Stress Reduction

Chair yoga offers a beautiful and accessible way to release tension and find solace from the stresses of daily life.

Practical Tips

1. **Create a Peaceful Space**: Find a quiet and comfortable space where you can practice without distractions.

2. **Mindful Presence**: Approach relaxation techniques with a gentle and open mindset. Allow yourself to fully engage in the present moment.

3. **Regular Practice**: Dedicate time each day to relaxation and stress relief techniques. Consistency is key to reaping the benefits.

Guided Relaxation Techniques

Guided relaxation techniques offer a pathway to deep relaxation and inner calm.

Practical Tips

1. **Softening Breath**: As you inhale, imagine drawing in a sense of calmness. As you exhale, release tension and stress.

2. **Body Scan**: Mentally scan your body from head to toe, relaxing each muscle group as you go along.

3. **Visualization**: Envision a peaceful place in your mind—a beach, a forest, or a garden. Immerse yourself in the sights, sounds, and sensations.

Gentle Stretches for Unwinding

Gentle stretches help release physical tension, providing a gateway to mental and emotional relaxation.

Practical Tips

1. **Ease into Stretches**: Approach each stretch with gentleness. Breathe deeply and gradually deepen the stretch without force.

2. **Mindful Movement**: Sync your breath with your stretches. Inhale to prepare, and exhale as you ease into the stretch.

3. **Focus on Breath**: Keep your attention on your breath as you stretch. Inhale to create space, and exhale to release tension.

Step-by-Step Instructions: Seated Relaxation and Forward Fold

1. **Sit comfortably:** on the edge of your chair with your feet flat on the floor and your hands resting on your legs.

2. **Relax Your Shoulders**: Inhale, roll your shoulders up to your ears, and exhale, letting them relax down your back.

3. **Inhale, Lift, and Lengthen**: Inhale deeply, lifting your chest and lengthening your spine.

4. **Exhale, Forward Fold**: Exhale, hinge forward from your hips, allowing your torso to gently descend toward your thighs.

5. **Relax Your Neck**: Let your head hang naturally, releasing any tension in your neck and shoulders.

6. **Breathe and Soften**: Take slow, deep breaths as you hold the stretch for 5-8 breaths. Feel your spine lengthening and your muscles releasing.

7. **Inhale and Rise**: Inhale, engage your core, and slowly roll back up to an upright seated position.

As you conclude this chapter, embrace the serenity that relaxation and stress relief techniques bring to your chair yoga practice. By consistently dedicating time to unwind and cultivate calmness, you are nurturing your mental and emotional well-being. In the upcoming chapter, we will wrap up our journey with insights on integrating chair yoga into your daily life, empowering you to continue reaping the benefits long after this program concludes.

Chapter 11: Chair-Assisted Standing Poses

Greetings and welcome to Chapter 11 of "28 Days of Chair Yoga for Seniors." In this chapter, we will embark on an exploration of chair-assisted standing poses, delving into the wonderful benefits they offer for leg strength, balance, and overall vitality. As an experienced yoga instructor with over 25 years of practice, I am excited to guide you through a series of practical exercises that will allow you to gradually transition from seated to standing postures with the support of a chair, empowering you to experience the joy of standing poses in a safe and accessible manner.

Chair-Assisted Standing Poses Unveiled

Chair-assisted standing poses bridge the gap between seated and traditional standing poses, providing stability and support.

Practical Tips

1. **Steady Chair Placement**: Ensure that your chair is placed on a stable surface, and the backrest is securely positioned for support.

2. **Mindful Progression**: Gradually work your way up from seated poses to chair-assisted standing poses, allowing your body to adapt and strengthen.

3. **Use of Chair for Balance**: The chair provides a reliable point of balance. Use it for support as

needed, gradually reducing reliance as your confidence grows.

Benefits of Chair-Assisted Standing Poses

Chair-assisted standing poses offer a multitude of benefits, including improved leg strength, enhanced balance, and increased mobility.

Practical Tips

1. **Engage Your Core**: Activate your core muscles to stabilize your spine and support your balance during standing poses.

2. **Mindful Breath**: Maintain steady and conscious breathing as you move through these poses. Inhale to prepare, and exhale to find stability.

3. **Feel the Ground**: Imagine roots extending from your feet into the ground, grounding you and enhancing your stability.

Gradually Transitioning to Chair-Assisted Standing Poses

Take a mindful journey from seated to standing, gradually building strength and confidence in your practice.

Practical Tips

1. **Warm-Up**: Engage in a gentle warm-up before attempting chair-assisted standing poses to prepare your body for the transition.

2. **Step-by-Step Progression**: Follow a step-by-step progression, moving from seated to partially supported standing poses with the chair.

3. **Modify and Adapt**: Modify the poses as needed to suit your comfort level. Use the chair as a guide, adjusting your stance and grip for stability.

Step-by-Step Instructions: Chair-Assisted Forward Fold

1. **Stand Tall**: Stand facing the chair, feet hip-width apart, and parallel. Place your direct the backrest for support.

2. **Inhale and Lengthen**: Inhale deeply, lengthening your spine upward. Feel the crown of your head reaching toward the ceiling.

3. **Exhale, Hinge Forward**: As you exhale, hinge forward from your hips, maintaining a long spine. Allow your hands to rest on the chair.

4. **Breathe and Lengthen**: Take slow, deep breaths as you hold the pose for 3-5 breaths. Feel the stretch in your hamstrings and lower back.

5. **Inhale and Rise**: Inhale, engage your core, and slowly rise back up to a standing position.

As you conclude this chapter, recognize the progress you are making in your chair-assisted standing poses. By embracing these exercises with mindfulness and patience, you are enhancing your leg strength, balance, and overall physical well-being. In the concluding chapter, we will reflect on your journey and offer insights on integrating chair yoga principles into your daily life for a lasting impact.

Chapter 12: Modified Sun Salutations

Greetings and welcome to Chapter 12, the concluding chapter, of "28 Days of Chair Yoga for Seniors." In this chapter, we will explore the adaptation of traditional sun salutations for chair yoga practice, creating a flowing sequence that will energize and invigorate your body while honoring your unique needs and capabilities. Drawing upon my extensive experience as a yoga instructor with over 25 years of practice, I am excited to guide you through a step-by-step process of a modified sun salutation routine, providing you with a wonderful way to integrate movement, breath, and mindfulness into your daily life.

The Essence of Modified Sun Salutations

Modified sun salutations offer a revitalizing and accessible way to engage in a classic yoga practice, tailored to your chair yoga journey.

Practical Tips

1. **Listen to Your Body**: Honor your body's signals. Modify and adapt the sequence as needed to ensure comfort and safety.

2. **Breath and Movement**: Sync your breath with each movement. Inhale as you expand, and exhale as you fold or contract.

3. **Flow Mindfully**: Move with intention and awareness. The focus is on creating a seamless connection between breath and movement.

Creating Your Chair Yoga Sun Salutation Sequence

Craft a sequence that honors the sun salutation tradition while embracing the chair yoga practice.

Practical Tips

1. **Adapt Poses**: Replace traditional poses with chair-assisted poses that mimic the essence of the movement.

2. **Modify Transitions**: Simplify transitions to accommodate seated and standing movements.

3. **Include Breath Awareness**: Infuse your sequence with mindful breathing. Use the breath to guide and enhance each movement.

Step-by-Step Instructions: Modified Chair Yoga Sun Salutation

Discover the beauty of a modified sun salutation routine, tailored to your chair yoga practice.

Practical Tips

1. **Warm-Up**: Engage in gentle warm-up movements for a few minutes to prepare your body.

2. **Mindful Breath**: Sync your breath with each movement. Inhale to expand, and exhale to contract.

3. **Seated Variations**: Adapt standing poses to seated versions, using the chair for support and balance.

Step-by-Step Instructions: Modified Chair Yoga Sun Salutation Sequence

1. **Seated Mountain Pose**: Sit tall on the edge of your chair, hands resting on your thighs. Inhale, lengthen your spine.

2. **Seated Forward Fold**: Exhale, hinge forward from your hips, reaching your hands toward the floor or chair legs.

3. **Seated Lunge**: Inhale, step your right foot back, creating a lunge position. Use the chair for support as needed.

4. **Seated Downward Dog**: Exhale, press your hands into the chair and lift your hips, creating an inverted V shape.

5. **Seated Upward Dog**: Inhale, shift forward into a modified plank, lowering your hips and lifting your chest.

6. **Seated Child's Pose**: Exhale, sit back on your heels, reaching your arms forward on the chair.

7. **Return to Seated Mountain**: Inhale, rise back up to seated mountain pose.

8. **Repeat on the Other Side**: Mirror the sequence, starting with your left foot for the seated lunge.

As you conclude this chapter and our 28-day journey, take a moment to reflect on the transformation you have experienced through chair yoga. By embracing this modified sun salutation and integrating the principles of chair yoga into your daily life, you are cultivating a deep connection between body, breath, and mind. Carry the essence of your practice with you, embracing movement, mindfulness, and well-being as you navigate your journey ahead. Thank you for joining me on this enriching exploration of chair yoga for seniors. Namaste.

Chapter 13: Upper Body Strength and Mobility

Greetings and welcome to Chapter 13 of "28 Days of Chair Yoga for Seniors." In this chapter, we will embark on a journey to enhance your upper body strength and flexibility through a series of chair-based exercises. By focusing on strengthening the arms, shoulders, and chest, we will work to improve functional fitness and support your overall well-being. Drawing upon my extensive experience as a yoga instructor with over 25 years of practice, I am excited to guide you through a variety of practical exercises, offering variations to cater to various levels of upper body strength.

The Importance of Upper Body Strength and Mobility

A strong and mobile upper body is essential for maintaining independence and participating fully in daily activities.

Practical Tips

1. **Gradual Progression**: Begin with exercises that suit your current level of strength and gradually work your way up to more challenging movements.

2. **Mind-Body Connection**: Focus on the sensations in your upper body during each exercise. Tune into the engagement of muscles and your breath.

3. **Safety First**: Maintain proper alignment and posture to prevent strain or injury. Use the chair for support as needed.

Chair-Based Upper Body Exercises

Chair-based exercises provide a safe and effective way to strengthen your upper body without the need for heavy weights or equipment.

Practical Tips

1. **Consistency is Key**: Dedicate a few minutes each day to upper body exercises for optimal results. Regular practice yields gradual improvements.

2. **Use of Props**: If needed, use props like a small cushion or resistance band to add variety and intensity to your exercises.

3. **Quality Over Quantity**: Focus on performing each exercise with proper form and control, rather than rushing through repetitions.

Variations for Different Levels of Strength

Explore a range of exercises with varying levels of intensity to accommodate various levels of upper body strength.

Practical Tips

1. **Beginner's Variation**: Start with basic exercises that involve minimal resistance, gradually building strength and confidence.

2. **Intermediate Variation**: Progress to exercises that involve slightly more resistance or challenge, as your strength increases.

3. **Advanced Variation**: Once you are comfortable with the intermediate exercises, explore more

advanced movements to further enhance your strength and mobility.

Step-by-Step Instructions: Chair-Assisted Push-Up

1. **Position Your Hands**: Sit on the edge of the chair, place your hands on the seat with your fingers pointing forward, and your thumbs pointing outward.

2. **Engage Your Core**: Inhale, engage your core muscles, and press through your hands to lift your hips off the chair.

3. **Lower Your Body**: Exhale, bend your elbows, and lower your body toward the chair in a controlled manner. Keep your elbows close to your sides.

4. **Push Back Up**: Inhale, press through your palms, and straighten your arms to return to the starting position.

5. **Repeat the Movement**: Perform 5-10 repetitions, focusing on steady breathing and proper alignment.

As you conclude this chapter, embrace the sense of empowerment that upper body strength and mobility bring to your chair yoga practice. By incorporating these practical exercises mindfully and consistently, you are enhancing your functional fitness and nurturing your overall physical well-being. Your journey through "28 Days of Chair Yoga for Seniors" has equipped you with valuable tools to support your health and vitality. Carry the wisdom of your practice with you as you continue your path of well-being.

Chapter 14: Gentle Inversions and Relaxing Poses

Greetings and welcome to Chapter 14 of "28 Days of Chair Yoga for Seniors." In this chapter, we will delve into the realm of gentle inversions and relaxing poses, exploring the transformative power of using a chair for support. We will discover the benefits of inversions for circulation and relaxation, and we will incorporate calming poses that promote a profound sense of well-being. Drawing upon my extensive experience as a yoga instructor with over 25 years of practice, I am delighted to guide you through a series of practical exercises and step-by-step instructions, allowing you to embrace the serenity and rejuvenation that gentle inversions and relaxing poses offer.

Embracing Gentle Inversions

Gentle inversions offer a unique perspective and a chance to enhance circulation and relaxation.

Practical Tips

1. **Chair Support**: Use the chair as a prop to facilitate safe and accessible inversions.

2. **Mindful Approach**: Approach inversions with patience and mindfulness. Listen to your body and proceed in a manner that is appropriate.

3. **Breath Awareness**: Maintain a steady and conscious breath throughout each inversion. Inhale to prepare, and exhale as you move into the pose.

Benefits of Inversions for Circulation and Relaxation

Inversions bring fresh blood flow to the brain, promoting relaxation and a sense of well-being.

Practical Tips

1. **Gentle Gradual Progression**: Start with slight inversions and gradually increase the angle as you become more comfortable.

2. **Relaxation Focus**: Embrace inversions as an opportunity to release tension and calm the mind.

3. **Safely Exit Poses**: Always exit inversions mindfully and with control, using the chair for support.

Incorporating Calming Poses

Discover a range of calming poses that offer relaxation and serenity.

Practical Tips

1. **Create a Tranquil Space**: Practice in a quiet and peaceful environment to enhance the calming effect of the poses.

2. **Extended Exhalation**: Lengthen your exhalation to enhance the relaxation response. Breathe deeply and fully.

3. **Soft Gaze**: Maintain a soft gaze or close your eyes during these poses to turn your focus inward.

Step-by-Step Instructions: Supported Legs Up the Chair

1. **Sit Close to the Chair**: Sit at the edge of the chair facing away from it, with your hips close to the seat.

2. **Lie Back**: Gently lie back on the floor, extending your legs up the seat of the chair.

3. **Supported Inversion**: Rest your legs on the chair, allowing your pelvis to lift slightly. Adjust your distance from the chair for comfort.

4. **Relax and Breathe**: Relax your arms by your sides, palms facing up. Close your eyes and take slow, deep breaths.

5. **Hold and Release**: Stay in the pose for 3-5 minutes, allowing gravity to gently stretch your hamstrings and promote relaxation.

6. **Exit Mindfully**: Bend your knees, roll to one side, and use your hands to help yourself sit up slowly.

As you conclude this chapter, embrace the serenity and renewal that gentle inversions and relaxing poses bring to your chair yoga practice. By integrating these exercises mindfully and consistently, you are enhancing your circulation, calming your mind, and nurturing your overall well-being. Your journey through "28 Days of Chair Yoga for Seniors" has empowered you with tools to support your health and vitality. Carry the peace and tranquility of your practice with you, fostering a sense of well-being in all aspects of your life.

Chapter 15: Creating Your Personal Chair Yoga Routine

Greetings and welcome to Chapter 15, the culmination of your transformative journey through "28 Days of Chair Yoga for Seniors." In this chapter, we will empower you to craft a personalized chair yoga routine that aligns with your unique needs, preferences, and aspirations. Drawing upon my extensive experience as a yoga instructor with over 25 years of practice, I am excited to guide you through the process of designing a balanced and sustainable chair yoga routine. Let us explore how to incorporate poses from previous chapters and discover practical tips for maintaining motivation and consistency in your chair yoga practice.

Designing Your Customized Chair Yoga Routine

Your personal chair yoga routine is a reflection of your individual goals and preferences.

Practical Tips

1. **Self-Assessment**: Reflect on your physical condition, areas of focus (such as flexibility, strength, or relaxation), and any specific needs or limitations.

2. **Poses from Previous Chapters**: Draw inspiration from poses introduced in previous chapters. Select movements that resonate with you and address your goals.

3. **Balanced Sequence**: Aim for a well-rounded routine that includes warm-ups, seated poses, standing poses, inversions, and relaxation techniques.

Crafting Your Chair Yoga Sequence

Create a flowing sequence that supports your well-being and can be easily integrated into your daily routine.

Practical Tips

1. **Warm-Up**: Begin with gentle warm-up movements to prepare your body for the practice ahead.

2. **Variations and Modifications**: Choose variations and modifications that suit your current level of practice. Adapt poses to your comfort and needs.

3. **Mindful Transitions**: Ensure smooth transitions between poses. Focus on your breath and maintain awareness of your body's movements.

Staying Motivated and Consistent

Maintaining a consistent chair yoga practice requires dedication and mindful approaches.

Practical Tips

1. **Set Realistic Goals**: Establish achievable goals for your practice. Celebrate small victories and milestones along the way.

2. **Create a Routine**: Dedicate a specific time each day for your chair yoga practice. Consistency is key to experiencing the benefits.

3. **Mindful Presence**: Approach each practice session with mindfulness and intention. Embrace the present moment and the gift of self-care.

Step-by-Step Guide: Your Personalized Chair Yoga Routine

1. **Warm-Up**: Begin with gentle seated stretches and spinal movements, as introduced in Chapter 4.

2. **Strength and Mobility**: Incorporate upper body strength exercises from Chapter 13 and hip and leg mobility poses from Chapter 7.

3. **Balance and Coordination**: Include balance-focused poses from Chapter 9 to enhance stability and body awareness.

4. **Sun Salutation Flow**: Create a modified sun salutation sequence as detailed in Chapter 12, energizing your body, and connecting breath with movement.

5. **Gentle Inversions and Relaxation**: Embrace supported inversions and relaxing poses from Chapter 14 to promote relaxation and tranquility.

6. **Breath and Mindfulness**: Conclude with breath-centered techniques from Chapter 3 to anchor your practice and bring a sense of inner calm.

As you embark on the creation of your personalized chair yoga routine, honor the progress you have made and the self-care journey you have undertaken. By integrating these principles into your daily life, you are cultivating a lasting foundation for health, vitality, and well-being. I commend you on your dedication and perseverance. May your chair yoga practice continue to enrich your life, fostering a harmonious connection between body, mind, and spirit. Namaste.

Conclusion: Embracing Chair Yoga for a Lifetime of Wellness

Congratulations on reaching the conclusion of "28 Days of Chair Yoga for Seniors." Your commitment and dedication to this journey have laid the foundation for a lifetime of wellness, strength, and happiness. As you reflect on the past 28 days, take a moment to acknowledge the progress you have made, the insights you have gained, and the positive impact chair yoga has had on your overall well-being.

Reflecting on Your Chair Yoga Journey

Over the course of these 28 days, you have embarked on a transformative path of self-discovery and self-care. You have embraced the wisdom of chair yoga, exploring a wide range of poses, movements, and techniques tailored to your unique needs and capabilities. Your dedication to practice has not only enhanced your physical body but has also nurtured a deeper connection between your body, breath, and mind.

Celebrating Your Achievements

As you look back, celebrate your achievements, both big and small. Perhaps you have noticed increased flexibility in your spine, a newfound sense of balance, or a greater sense of calm and relaxation. These achievements are a testament to your commitment and the power of chair yoga to promote holistic well-being.

Continuing Your Chair Yoga Journey

Your journey with chair yoga does not end here—it is a lifelong practice that can continue to evolve and enrich your life. As you move forward, consider these words of encouragement:

1. **Stay Curious**: Keep exploring the world of chair yoga. There are endless possibilities to deepen your practice and explore new variations.

2. **Listen to Your Body**: Your body is your greatest guide. Tune in to its signals and adjust your practice to honor its needs and limitations.

3. **Consistency Matters**: Consistency is the key to reaping the benefits of chair yoga. Dedicate time each day to your practice, no matter how brief.

4. **Mindful Living**: Carry the mindfulness and presence you have cultivated on the mat into your daily life. Use your breath and awareness to navigate challenges and find moments of tranquility.

5. **Community and Support**: Consider joining a chair yoga class or connecting with fellow practitioners to share experiences and insights.

Remember that chair yoga is a tool you can always turn to—a source of strength, balance, and rejuvenation. Your journey is a lifelong partnership between you and your body, and chair yoga is here to support you every step of the way.

As you conclude this program, I extend my deepest gratitude for allowing me to be a part of your chair yoga journey. May your path be filled with health, joy, and a profound sense of well-being. Keep breathing, keep moving, and keep embracing the gift of chair yoga. Namaste.

www.ingramcontent.com/pod-product-compliance
Lightning Source LLC
Chambersburg PA
CBHW050853260726
48660CB00006B/2608